Nutritious Diet During Pregnancy:

A Must For Delivering
A Healthy Birth Weight Baby

BECKY FLYNN

Disclaimer and Terms of Use:

The Author and Publisher has strived to be as accurate and complete as possible in the creation of this book, notwithstanding the fact that he/she does not warrant or represent at any time that the contents within are accurate due to the rapidly changing nature of the Internet. While all attempts have been made to verify information provided in this publication, the Author and Publisher assumes no responsibility for errors, omissions, or contrary interpretation of the subject matter herein. Any perceived slights of specific persons, peoples, or organizations are unintentional. This book is not intended for use as a source of legal, business, accounting or financial advice. All readers are advised to seek services of competent professionals in legal, business, health, accounting, and finance field. Please consult with your Physician before taking any medical advice.

Table of Contents

Introduction

When you are pregnant one of the most important things that you can do is to eat healthy. A woman who eats healthy when she is pregnant is more likely to not only deliver a healthy baby, but the delivery process itself will go much smoother if she has eaten well through her entire pregnancy. Many women can attest that the labor process can be very difficult and can consist of hours upon hours of contractions. Not to mention just how being pregnant itself takes a huge toll on a woman's body. Thus eating healthy before you become pregnant and when you become pregnant is essential to providing yourself with the energy that you need to make it through the pregnancy.

Research has shown that a woman who eats healthy when she has become pregnant have a safe and uncomplicated pregnancy. Eating healthy is not only important for a woman before she is pregnant, but also after she delivers the baby. The baby will need all of the nutrients that it can get it after it comes into this world. It should be a woman's goal to continue to eat healthy after she delivers. Eating healthy after delivery is also a good idea, as it will allow her to have the energy she needs to take care of her new child.

Throughout this book we will cover the topics that are associated with eating healthy when you are pregnant. Such as what foods you should eat and when you should eat them. What foods have the maximum amount of nutrients and how you can take advantage of those foods when you are pregnant. What is a healthy amount of weight to gain when you are pregnant? How eating well really does affect the health of your baby? Also what dietary supplements you should be eating. This book will cover all of those subjects and more. You will then understand why it is necessary for you to eat healthy while you are pregnant.

Eating To Conceive

Before a woman conceives it is important that she first visits with her doctor. Why she needs to visit with her doctor first is to ensure that she is healthy enough to withstand the challenges of being pregnant. A doctor will be able tell her if she needs to gain or lose weight in order to become pregnant. He can also do a physical and make sure that there is nothing that might prevent her from becoming pregnant. A doctor might recommend any number of things, from totally changing her diet to starting an exercise program. A doctor is the most valuable source of information to a woman when she is pregnant. A pregnant woman should consult frequently with her doctor throughout the term of the pregnancy.

The first thing a woman should do when she is pregnant is to stop eating unhealthy foods. Unhealthy food choices such as that morning coffee or that afternoon coke are good places to start. A pregnant woman should begin to cut out all caffeine and sugar from her diet.

Caffeine is a stimulant and is not healthy for a pregnant woman to have. Caffeine is known to be a reason for miscarriages. Sugar should be cut out of the diet because it destroys the immune system. Both can increase the chances of having a miscarriage. If a woman smokes she should most definitely stop smoking. Smoking is also another factor that greatly increases the chance of a miscarriage.

It is recommended that a woman starts eating healthy long before she is pregnant This diet should include eating fruits and vegetables as well as a high protein diet that includes eggs and meats. All foods consumed when pregnant should contain a very high nutritional value. Any food that is green is a must in a pregnant woman's diet. You will want to begin adding foods into your diet that are rich in folic acid. Eating oranges and drinking a lot of orange juice is a very good idea as they contain high values of folic acid. Strawberries, beans, beats and nuts also contain folic acid.

Folic acid supports the placenta as well as prevents spina bifda and other neural tube defects. Foods with folic acid should be eaten while a woman is trying to get pregnant because it cleans the correct tubs that are necessary for her to get pregnant. No doubt folic acid should be consumed when a woman is pregnant as well. However, it is especially important while a woman is trying to get pregnant.

A pregnant woman should also be taking vitamins and supplements to add to her nutritional intake. These vitamins should be taken when a woman is pregnant: C, D, B as well as vitamins B6 and B12. Supplements such as calcium, iron and zinc should also be considered.

When you are pregnant water should always be the first drink of choice. Next to water a pregnant woman should be drinking pasteurized fruit juices. Milk should also be drank as a source of calcium.

Getting pregnant should not be taken lightly. You should take all of the necessary procedures to ensure that it goes well. Remember that when you are pregnant you are not only taking care of yourself, but you are also taking care of another human that is inside of you. The proper nutrition will ensure that both you and the baby will live a long and a healthy life.

Basics Of Eating Healthy
When Pregnant

So lets overview some of the general things regarding what to eat when you are pregnant. We will then cover some more subjects about staying healthy when you are pregnant.

You will need at least three servings a day of protein. This can be gotten by eating three servings of fruit or drinking several glasses of apple juice every day. Eating a serving or two of yogurt a day is also a good choice.

Calcium is very important when you are pregnant. You need to have at least four servings of calcium a day. This Calcium intake can be either through supplements or by drinking three glasses of milk a day. This can also be achieved through the occasional ice cream treat.

Vitamin C is also very important for a pregnant woman. A pregnant woman should have at least three servings of Vitamin C a day. Again this can be done in the form of supplements or in drinking two or three glasses of orange juice a day.

Three or four servings of fruit and vegetables a day are a must as this will keep you functioning at your prime level.

Iron is one supplement that your body really needs. The longer that you are pregnant the greater your body's need for iron will become. It is important to take iron supplements on a daily basis. You should consult your doctor to determine just how much iron that your body needs in order to be functioning at its prime level.

Eating healthy and staying healthy is the foundation of health for both you are your baby. That is why it is vital that you keep yourself and your baby healthy.

This is what the diet of a pregnant woman should look like on a day to day basis. Note this is just an example.

Breakfast
1 Serving of fruit salad
¼ Cup of cottage cheese topping
1 Low-fat oatmeal muffin
1 Cup of 1% milk

Snack
1 Oz. of cheese
4 to 6 whole grain crackers

Lunch
1 Serving of beef fajita salad
1 Kiwi

Snack
3 Cups of air-popped popcorn
¼ Cup of shredded light cheddar for topping

Dinner
1 Serving of chickpea and broccoli curry
1 Serving of full of folate salad

Mixed berry fruit salad
½ Cup fresh or frozen unsweetened berries
Dash of almond extract
½ Cup of low-fat yogurt

Snack
1 Cup of bran cereal
½ Cup of 1% milk

Source: www.todaysparent.com/images/foodnutrition/tp
-preg-meal-plan.pdf

A pregnant woman should increase her calorie intake by 150 calories at the beginning of the pregnancy and be eating 300-500 more calories by the end of her pregnancy.

A woman should also increase her protein intake while she is pregnant. A daily intake of bread, fruit or pasta is needed for a healthy pregnancy. Fats are also necessary for the development of the baby's nervous system.

Below is a basic chart that you should consider following to ensure that you are getting all of the vitamins that you need.

Essential Vitamin/Mineral:	Why You Need It:	Where You Find It:
Vitamin A &Beta Carotene (770 mcg)	Helps bones and teeth grow	Liver, milk, eggs, carrots, spinach, green and yellow vegetables, broccoli, potatoes, pumpkin, yellow fruits, cantaloupe
Vitamin D (5 mcg)	Helps body use calcium and phosphorus; promotes strong teeth and bones	Milk, fatty fish, sunshine
Vitamin E (15 mg)	Helps body form and use red blood cells and muscles	Vegetable oil, wheat germ, nuts, spinach, fortified cereals
Vitamin C (80 - 85 mg)	An antioxidant that protects tissues from damage and helps body absorb iron; builds a healthy immune system	Citrus fruits, bell peppers, green beans, strawberries, papaya, potatoes, broccoli, tomatoes
Thiamin/B1 (1.4 mg)	Raises the energy level and regulates nervous system	Whole grain, fortified cereals, wheat germ, organ meats, eggs, rice, pasta, berries, nuts, legumes, pork
Riboflavin/B2 (1.4 mg)	Maintains energy, good eyesight, healthy skin	Meats, poultry, fish, dairy products, fortified cereals, eggs
Niacin/B3 (18 mg)	Promotes healthy skin, nerves and digestion	High-protein foods, fortified cereals and breads, meats, fish, milk, eggs, peanuts
Pyridoxine/B6 (1.9 mg)	Helps form red blood cells; helps with morning sickness	Chicken, fish, liver, pork, eggs, soybeans, carrots, cabbage, cantaloupe, peas, spin-

		ach, wheat germ, sunflower seeds, bananas, beans, broccoli, brown rice, oats, bran, peanuts, walnuts
Folic Acid/Folate (600 mcg)	Helps support the placenta, and prevents spina bifida and other neural tube defects	Oranges, orange juice, strawberries, green leafy vegetables, spinach, beets, broccoli, cauliflower, fortified cereals, peas, pasta, beans, nuts
Calcium (1,000 - 1,300 mg)	Creates strong bones and teeth, helps prevent blood clots, helps muscles and nerve function	Yogurt, milk, cheddar cheese, calcium-fortified foods like soy milk, juices, breads, cereals, dark green leafy vegetables, canned fish with bones
Iron (27 mg)	Helps in the production of hemoglobin; prevents anemia, low birth weight, and premature delivery	Beef, pork, dried beans, spinach, dried fruits, wheat germ, oatmeal or grains fortified with iron
Protein (71 mg)	Helps in the production of amino acids; repairs cells	Most animal foods, meat, poultry, eggs, dairy products, veggie burgers, beans, legumes, nuts
Zinc (11-12 mg)	Helps produce insulin and enzymes	Red meats, poultry, beans, nuts, whole grains, fortified cereals, oysters, dairy products

Resourced from: www.americanpregnancy.org/pregnancyhealth/nutrientsvitaminspregnancy.html

At this point we are going to cover the different trimesters. As a woman you need to understand each stage of the pregnancy and how eating right really can effect things throughout your pregnancy.

The First Trimester

Conception typically occurs two weeks after your period. Doctors will often calculate your due date from the date of your first period. The conception period typically last one or two weeks.

The third week is when fertilization happens. This is when the egg and sperm unite and form what is called one cell. If more than one cell is released then this is when you can have twins.

These groups of cells them begin their journey towards the uterus. The inner most group of cells will begin to form into the embryo. While the outer most groups of cells will begin to nourish and protect the most inner group of cells.

These cells when then begin to implant into the uterine wall for both nourishment and protection. That is why this phase is called implementation.

Five weeks into the pregnancy mark the beginning of the embryonic period. This period will start to lay the foundation for the circulatory system. By the time the fifth week is finished your baby will start to take shape and be about as small as the tip of an ink pen.

The sixth week is when your baby's neural tube closes. After this happens your baby really begins to start taking shape. The arms and the legs will begin to appear at this stage. At this point the heart of the baby begins pumping blood on its own as well.

Seven weeks into the pregnancy your baby's head starts to really take shape. This of course also means that the brain of your baby is beginning to develop.

The eighth week into the pregnancy is when the eyes of the baby become visible. At this point the baby's body also begins to rapidly develop. The arms and the legs begin to grow visibility longer and the trunk of the baby's body is starting to form.

Nine weeks into the pregnancy the baby's toes begin to take shape. At this point your baby's body is making huge progress and is starting to grow by leaps and bounds.

By the tenth week your baby's neck is starting to develop. Its head is also starting to take shape and starting to form into a round shape.

By week 10 and 11 the baby's genitals begin to form. As well as it's fingernails.

This concludes the first trimester of the pregnancy.

The Second Trimester

Thirteen weeks into the pregnancy your baby's umbilical cord begins to form. The tissue that will become bone is starting to develop in your baby's body. This tissue begins to develop around your baby's head, as well as its arms and legs.

The fourteenth week is when your baby's sex becomes apparent. At this point your baby is about 3 ½ inches long. The baby's red blood cells also begin to form in the spleen area.

The fifteenth week is when the baby's skeleton and bones will begin to develop. The baby's hair pattern will also begin to develop around this week as well.

By the sixteenth week your baby will begin to make sucking motions. You might not be able to feel your baby's movements at this time, but an ultrasound will be able to detect slight movements of the baby.

The seventeenth week of the pregnancy is when fat stores will begin to develop underneath your baby's skin. This fat will keep your baby warm after it is born.

Eighteen weeks into the pregnancy is when your baby begins to hear. It is possible that your baby could be 5 ½ inches long by this time as well.

Nineteen weeks into the pregnancy is when a greasy like substance begins to cover your baby's body. This will protect your baby's skin from the amniotic fluid.

At week twenty of the pregnancy you might be able to feel the baby's movements inside of you. Week twenty is also the halfway point in the pregnancy. At this time your baby could be a little longer than 6 inches.

The twenty-first week the baby is becoming much more active in the womb and you are really starting to feel the baby's movements. At this time the baby can also swallow.

The twenty-second week of the pregnancy the baby's hair can be seen on the ultrasound. It is also possible your baby's eyebrows will become visible. At this time it is very possible that your baby is 7 ½ inches long.

The twenty-third week of the pregnancy your baby will be able to start moving its eyes. Its tastes buds will also begin to develop. At this time the baby might be formed enough so that it will have actual finger prints.

The twenty-fourth week the baby could be 8 inches or longer and is rapidly growing.

By the twenty-fifth week the baby's hearing is good enough to be able to respond to the sound of your voice.

The twenty-sixth week is when the baby starts to grow its fingernails. It is also during this time the baby's lungs begin to inflate. The baby's lungs start to produce a surfactant. This substance allows the baby's lungs to inflate and deflate without sticking together.

Week twenty-seven is when the baby's is really growing. The mother will begin to feel the baby move more and more. This week also ends the second trimester and begins the third trimester.

The Third Trimester

The twenty-eighth week the baby's eyes begin to open. At this point your baby could be about 10 inches long and now the baby is going to start gaining weight. The baby at this point could weigh more than 2 pounds.

The twenty-ninth week of the pregnancy is the week when the baby's bones are fully developed. They are still soft at this point, but they are fully developed.

By week thirty the baby's eyes are open most of the time. The red blood cells have now formed in the baby's bone marrow. Your baby at this point could weigh more than 3 pounds and be more than 10 ½ inches long.

The thirty-first week the baby has matured enough to where it can control its own body temperature.

The thirty-second week the baby's fingernails and toe-nails are now visible. The baby is also now almost totally breathing on its own.

The thirty-third week the baby's pupils can at last detect light.

In the last few weeks of pregnancy many things begin to occur. By the thirty-fourth week the baby could be nearly 12 inches long. The baby's fingernails are now also fully grown.

The thirty-fifth week things continue to progress and your baby continues to gain weight.

The thirty-sixth week you are more than likely going to start feeling the baby a lot moving around inside of you. The baby is gaining a lot of weight during this season.

The thirty-seventh week is when the baby is fully grown and the baby could at this point turn its head to start the position it will be in when it is going to be in labor.

From week thirty-eight to forty the baby continues to grow and reaches 18-20 inches in length and the baby's weight grows from six and a half pounds all of the way to nine pounds. Then, sometime during the fortieth week the mother gives birth to her baby.

How To Prune Yourself
Off A Bad Diet

There are many things you can do to wean yourself off bad food if you are an expecting mother. The first thing you need to do is to consider your blood sugar. Most junk foods tend to increase your blood sugar because of their carbohydrate and sugar levels. If you are craving junk food you should eat a few chocolate chips instead of eating an entire chocolate chip cookie.

Your hunger could be because your blood sugar levels are low. This is why it is good to never skip meals. Eating six times a day should keep this from happening. When you get extremely hungry you will be more prone to eat junk food.

The best way to stop craving junk food is to start eating healthy. The nutrition that you attain when you are eating healthy will help to ease most of your junk food cravings.

If you do find yourself craving sugar it is best to avoid any artificial sweeteners. Several studies have shown that artificial sweeteners will only increase your sugar cravings. Artificial sweeteners are also known to cause cancer.

Emotional triggers can set you towards eating foods with high sugar content. It is best to learn what triggers you to eat foods that have a high sugar content. When you learn what triggers you to eat junk food you can easily manage not only your emotions, but also your food intake.

There are certain diets that you can follow that will allow you wean yourself off high carbohydrate and sugary diets. It is best to be weaned off junk food before you get pregnant.

Many women who continue to eat junk food during their pregnancy will have delivery room issues. They are prone to deliver the baby before the baby is due. They also will have many complications after the baby is born.

Gestational Diabetes

Gestational diabetes is one of the most common pregnancy complications that women face. Gestational diabetes is when women have high blood sugar levels when they are pregnant. There are basically two treatments for Gestational diabetes. The first one is an insulin shot. However the only true cure for it is to deliver the baby. Usually after the baby is delivered a woman's blood sugar level will return back to normal.

If you do happen to develop gestational diabetes your doctor will refer you to a nutritionist. The nutritionist will have you spread out your sugar and carbohydrate intake. However, one of the best things that you can do is to give up sugar entirely. The nutritionist will also encourage you to go on a low carb diet for the rest of your pregnancy. You will also be strongly encouraged to not skip any meals.

If you are diagnosed with Gestational diabetes you will have to check your blood sugar levels on a regular basis. Not doing these things could put you at risk for developing diabetes later on in life. However the greater the risk will be for the child that you are carrying. Not getting your blood sugar level under control could very well be putting the child you are carrying at risk, as well as your own.

If your child is larger than normal and you have Gestational Diabetes the chances that you will have a C-section or have delivery issues will greatly increase.

This is one of the primary reasons why both doctors and nutritionist alike say that you should get your diet under control long before you become pregnant to avoid all of these issues.

Food That Should be Avoided When Pregnant

Foods that should be avoided when pregnant are also foods that everyone should avoid in most cases. For example raw meat should be avoided for the obvious reasons.

However some other foods should be avoided that you might not think of. Food products that are made from unpasteurized milk should be avoided. This includes some cheeses such as feta and gorgonzola. The reason for this is unpasteurized milk products contain listeria. Raw eggs should be stayed away from and anything that contains them such as cookie dough.

Other foods are debatable as to what should and should not be eaten when a woman is pregnant. Fish is up to debate. Some nutritional professionals say it is perfectly fine for a woman to eat fish when she is pregnant. Others say that women should stay away from all fish because of the risk of mercy poising.

This is a basic list of foods that should be avoided or questioned when you are pregnant.

• Deli Meat: May contain listeria

• Fish: May contain high levels of Mercy and may be exposed to industrial pollutants

• Smoked Seafood: May contain listeria

• Raw Eggs: May contain salmonella

• Soft Cheeses: May contain listeria

• Unpasteurized milk: May contain listeria

• Caffeine: Caffeine intake may be related to miscarriages

• Alcohol: May cause Fetal Alcohol Syndrome. No amount of Alcohol is safe when pregnant.

• All fruits and vegetables should be thoroughly washed to avoid exposure to toxoplasmosis

Eating To Prevent Heartburn

Heartburn is a common condition that pregnant women face. The reason is that your baby has grown a tremendous amount and your uterus has moved up and is now putting pressure on your stomach. This crowds the digestive tract and allows acids to travel back up to the esophagus. It is estimated that one in four women will suffer from heartburn when they are pregnant. Thus it is a very common condition. There are a few ways to prevent or to at the very least lessen this condition.

One the best things that you can do is to have an early dinner. Eating two or three hours before you go to bed will greatly decrease your chance of getting heartburn. Another good thing you can do to prevent heartburn it is to be a slow eater. Eating slowly will allow a nice amount for your food to digest and prevent heartburn. Most doctors recommend that pregnant women should eat six meals a day. What this means is that you should eat three large meals and three snacks between each meal. Your large meals should be smaller meals as you will be eating plenty of snacks between your meals.

When you eat, your fluids should be separate from your meals. Food and fluid mixed together can irritate your stomach. Doctors recommend that normal people keep their meals and fluids separate. When you are pregnant it is especially important to keep these separate to avoid the risk of getting heartburn.

When you eat your meals it is important that you are in an upright position. It is never a good idea to eat while you are laying down when you are pregnant.

If you are a heavy person you might be more prone to experience heartburn when you are pregnant verses say if you are a smaller and lighter person. Thus if you want to avoid heartburn when you are pregnant you should lose some weight.

When you are pregnant all hot and spicy foods should be avoided to prevent the onset of heartburn.

Heartburn might not be able to ever be totally avoided when you are pregnant, but there are plenty of things that can be done in order to prevent it.

Food Cravings

Food cravings are nutritionally based. Thus if your body needs some nutrient then your body will crave that nutrient. It is estimated that 68% of women will experience food cravings at some point during her pregnancy. Sometimes food cravings can even be the first indicator of if you are having a boy or a girl. If you are craving sweets then you very well could be having a girl. If you are craving meats and other similar food then you could very well be having a boy.

There are a few ways to prevent some of the crazy food cravings that women get when they are pregnant. A healthy breakfast is always a good idea. The higher the nutritional value of the food that you are eating the less food cravings that you will have.

However even eating the healthiest foods will not prevent the crazy food cravings that you will get when you are pregnant. Honesty, sometime it is better to just give into the cravings. There is nothing wrong with not eating healthy every so often as long as you do not make a habit of it. If you are craving pizza or chocolate a lot there is nothing wrong with eating it in small portions to ease or even prevent future food cravings like that.

Your goal when pregnant should be eating as healthy as possible. However moderation is important and there is nothing wrong with caving into your cravings every so often.

Food Aversions

Food aversions are the exact opposite of food cravings. Food aversions and food cravings happen to nearly every woman that is pregnant. A food aversion is to really not want a food that you would typically want to eat.

A food craving could very well be a way of telling your body that you need to eat a certain food. A food aversion could be a way of telling your body telling you that you do not need a certain food.

Food aversions are known for triggering what is normally called morning sickness. Most food aversions start in the first trimester of pregnancy, but end by the second trimester. Some woman complain of food aversions lasting the entire pregnancy. However, this is very uncommon.

You should not try to avoid food aversions. Many times they are a sign that you should not be eating the food that you are having the food aversion to. If you have food aversions for healthy foods then you might want to consider fighting the aversion. Your body needs healthy food more than anything else at this time in your life.

Maybe you are having a food aversion to fruits. Instead of eating fruits you can get a juicer and juice your fruits so you are drinking them instead of eating them.

There is a number of ways to deal with food aversions. Most importantly realize that you are pregnant and give yourself some grace. Food aversions are normal and you can handle them as they come.

Nausea and Vomiting In Pregnancy

There is no known cause for morning sickness. However, some doctors have several ideas of what causes morning sickness. Morning sickness primarily is just going to happen in the first trimester of the pregnancy.

The first reason could be because of hormones rising in the woman's system because of the pregnancy. Studies have shown that nausea tends to peak around the time that hormone and estrogen levels are rising or beginning to peak.

During the first trimester pregnant women have an enhanced sense of smell. Thus they become more sensitive to many more things. This causes there reflexes to be enhanced and this also cause nausea and vomiting.

A woman's stomach is also much more sensitive when she is pregnant and this is another reason why she is more prone to vomit.

Most doctors agree that one of the best ways to avoid morning sickness is to eat food that is naturally made. Thus avoid all prepackaged and processed products. Why doctors recommend this is because most women will not get the proper nutrition that they need when they eat foods that nature does not produce.

There is no way to end morning sickness. Even while eating a proper diet you will more than likely suffer through episodes of morning sickness.

Constipation and Pregnancy

As with all symptoms of pregnancy there is a reason for constipation. When you are pregnant your body creates progesterone which in turns relaxes the muscles of the bowels and causes your digestive tracks to work much slower. Your digestive track works slower to make sure your body absorb the nutrients from your food for your baby. This can create constipation, which if it not kept under control, can lead to hemorrhoids.

There are several things that can be done for this. The first thing is to stay active. Do not become a couch potato just because you are pregnant.

The next thing is to make sure that you have plenty of fluids flowing through your entire body. Stay well hydrated and drink at least 8-12 glasses of water every day.

It is also important to keep fiber going through your body. Thus it is important to eat a lot of fruits. Plums are an excellent source of fiber and have been a natural constipation reliever for a long time. If you cannot handle eating normal fruits all of the time because of the acid content then you could always eat dried fruits.

You should avoid eating food that can lead to constipation. This can include things like eating a lot of bread products. Also drinking milk can constipate some people. Stay away from foods that you know will cause you to have constipation problems. Eat food that has a high fiber content and drink plenty of water and you should be fine.

Healthy Weight Gain For A Pregnancy

Many doctors will tell you that you should gain between 25-30 pounds when you are pregnant. Most of this weight will occur in the second and third trimesters of a pregnancy. It is possible that you can lose weight your first trimester. The reason for this would be morning sickness. Your first trimester you should gain no more than 5 pounds.

During your second trimester you will probably gain between 12-15 pounds. This weight could come in phases. The longer that you are into your second trimester the more weight you will gain. If you are not gaining weight in your second trimester then you need to visit with your doctor.

You will gain most of your weight when you enter into your third trimester. At this point you could gain as much as one or two pounds per week. However towards the end of this time the weight could slow down some. Your eighth month of being pregnant is when you will put on the most weight.

The baby will at most weigh between eight and nine pounds. So where is the rest of the weight coming from? Let's examine that figure for a little while. The fluid that your baby has been swimming in can weigh up to two or three pounds. Your body is producing up to 4 or 5 pounds of extra blood because of the nature of the pregnancy. Finally by the time the baby is born your body could have produced an extra 9 or 10 pounds fat. That is why it is possible to weigh as much as 30 pounds more by the time your pregnancy is completed.

If you find that you are gaining a lot more weight than these numbers above then you probably need to be getting more exercise. If you find that you are not gaining these numbers at all then you probably need to be adding more calories to your diet. If your morning sickness is extremely bad this could also allow you to not gain the weight stated in this book. At last resort visit your doctor if you feel that you are gaining weight either too slow or too fast. A medical professional will be able to give you professional advice as to what action you need to take if any.

Diet and Mood Swings During Pregnancy

Most women are going to be more moody during the first and third trimesters. The first trimester you are going to be very tired as your body is going to be learning how to give both you and the baby the proper nutrition that you both need. You also will be putting up with a lot of morning sickness your first trimester. In your third trimester you are going to be dealing with gaining a lot of weight and will have difficulty sleeping because of this extra weight in addition to putting up with a constantly strained and sore body.

The physical changes of being pregnant will be strenuous enough. You are also going to be going through some emotional challenges since you will be bringing a new child into this world. It will be very important for you rest as much as possible when you are pregnant.

It is also important to remember that your mood swings are related to hormonal changes that are happening in your body. It is important to find friends and family that will support you at this time in your life. You will need all of the support that you can get.

Maintaining a healthy diet is a very important part of a healthy pregnancy. It is equally important to maintain a healthy emotional diet as well. Remember that your friends and family are there to support you.

Exercise and Pregnancy

Regular exercise when you are pregnant is a good idea for many women. It will help you maintain a high energy level. Exercise does get increasingly harder the further you get into your pregnancy. The first trimester is indeed the best time to maintain a regular exercise routine.

Many doctors and nutritionist highly recommend that you have an exercise routine for the entire time that you are pregnant. It will not only increase your energy level, but it will also aid in controlling any weight that you are putting on during your pregnancy. Many women and doctors say that it also helps in the delivery room.

If you do begin to do an exercise routine when you are pregnant there are several things that you need to keep an eye on. In some cases these things could end your exercise routine, but in most cases you should be fine.

If your heart rate is too high it could cause damage to your baby. Your goal should be to maintain a steady heart rate throughout your exercise process. If it rises too high or drops too low then you need to stop and come up with another game plan.

You should never start a totally new routine of exercising when you are pregnant. It is best to stay with a routine that you already know and have a good concept of. This is important because it will keep your body comfortable.

Walking is the most recommended form of exercise. It is something that you can do for all three trimesters of your pregnancy. Many women who walk have found that it makes delivering their baby much easier. Doctors recommend that you walk up until your due date to increase the chances of an easy delivery.

There are some cases that you should not exercise when you are pregnant. Below are some cases when you should not exercise.

• If you have had a history of giving birth to a premature baby.

• If you have any bleeding or spotting you should stop exercising immediately.

• If you have a history of having a low placenta or a weak cervix then you should not be exercising when you are pregnant.

The American Pregnancy Association has released some guidelines that you should follow when you are exercising. They are as follows.

• It is recommended that you start an exercise program very slowly if you are pregnant

• Always listen to your body. Your body will give you the proper signals of what to do and how to do it.

• Never exercise to the point of exhaustion.

• Wear Comfortable exercise support that provides you ankle and arch support.

• Take frequent breaks and drink plenty of water

• Avoid exercise in extremely hot weather.

• Avoid rocky terrain or unstable ground.

• Contact sports should be avoided.

• Avoid lifting weights above your head.

• During second and third trimesters avoid lying flat on your back as it decreases blood flow to your uterus.

• Include a relaxation and stretching program

• Eat a healthy diet that has plenty of fruits and vegetables.

Source: www.americanpregnancy.org/pregnancyhealth/exerciseguidelines.html

Food Allergies and Pregnancy

Because of what one eats and drinks can affect the baby either positively or adversely it is best to eliminate all foods that you are allergic too long before you ever become pregnant. The most common food allergy is a peanut food allergy.

If you have ever had to deal with any food allergy's then you would not want to put your child though those similar problems. It is a well known fact that almost everything in the grocery store nowadays has some form or fashion of either peanuts or peanut oil.

That is not to say that you should never eat peanuts when you are pregnant. Peanut butter does have a lot of the necessary protein in it that your body needs.

However if you have ever had any type of food allergy before, be that to peanuts or any other type of food then it is best to lay off that food while you are pregnant. At the very least consult a doctor before you get pregnant and ask them about food allergies and how to deal with them.

Vegetarians and Pregnancy

A vegetarian can have a healthy baby. There will be some steps that a vegetarian will have to take that a normal person might not even think of, but the main thing that a vegetarian will have to worry about is ensuring that the baby gets all of the protein that it needs.

The vegetarian will need to eat a lot more nuts than a non-vegetarian. Basically a vegetarian needs to eat food that has protein in it. Most protein is found in meat products. Fruits and vegetables also have a lot of protein in them as well. Thus Vegetarians need to eat a lot of fruits and vegetables, as well as a lot of nuts. It is very important that the protein that a non-vegetarian would get in meat is made up for in the vegetarian for the sake of the baby's health.

A Vegetarian might need to eat more than non-vegetarians to make up for the lack of protein.

The vegetarian should follow the same regiment as non-vegetarians as far as vitamin intake and proper amount of calorie intake.

The naysayers that say that a vegetarian cannot get pregnant are wrong. A vegetarian can have a healthy pregnancy and a healthy baby as long as they make up for the protein that they would normally get from eating meats.

Fetal Health Can Last A Lifetime

Throughout this book we have covered the necessities of eating healthy when you are pregnant. We have covered almost every area there is to be covered regarding eating and staying healthy when you are pregnant. From the basics of what you should and should not eat, all of the way to covering things like how much you should exercise and it is okay to be a vegetarian and get pregnant. Why we have taken the time to cover all of these issues is because when the fetus is in the womb it is setting up the health of the child for its entire life.

There have been numerous studies that have been done that tracked the health of a person back to the time when they were a fetus. For example a recent study that has been done has shown that infants that were born with a very low birth weight have an increased risk of glucose intolerance and could have an increased risk of coronary heart disease later on in life. It is also interesting to note that recent studies have shown that those who were born small often become large later in life. It is a well known fact that many overweight people have heart disease.

One must ask if a child is born underweight was the mother really taking care of herself when she was pregnant? It is true that in many third world countries it is nearly impossible for mothers to take care of themselves as they need to. However in many industrialized countries women have no excuse not to take proper care of themselves and give their future child all of the proper nutrition that he or she will need while they are still in the womb.

It is a scientific fact that healthy mothers have healthy babies. It is also a proven fact that sick mothers have sick baby's. In third world countries where many future mothers are already facing malnutrition, they produce babies that are underweight and have many different kinds of health problems.

There has been numerous studies that have been done that show how our health is programmed into us when we are a fetus. What a mother eats when she is pregnant can leave an imprint that can indeed last a lifetime. It has been proven in many studies that baby's that are born small could struggle with health problems for their entire lives. Most baby's that are born small will have mothers that have not taken care of their nutritional health or they will have been born too early.

Many mothers will try to overfeed a child that is born small. This will only work against what is called the baby's programming. Babies need to be fed a healthy and nutritious diet from birth. Trying to overfeed an underweight baby could increase the chance that the baby will become overweight later in life.

Did you know that if a mother is stressed, the baby the mother is carrying will also be stressed. That is just one more factor to consider. If a mother is eating a healthy diet and getting plenty of exercise she will just naturally be less stressed. Thus the baby will also be less stressed.

As many studies that have shown that if a baby is born smaller it can lead to an unhealthy life. There have been other studies that have been done that prove that a baby that is born healthy that they will lead a healthy life.

What happens to the baby when it is in the mothers womb could indeed affect the baby for its entire life. Good nutrition really does start in the womb. That is why it is vital for a future mother to not only be healthy before she is going to get pregnant, but also to continue to keep making the right food choices while she is pregnant.

We will cover later in this book the proper diet for a woman after she gives birth. A mother should continue to eat healthy long after she gives birth as she will nurse the baby.

Special Needs Pregnancy

This is a topic that is not covered in most books. However I feel that it is an important topic to cover. There is a special screening that is done between the 15th and 18th weeks of pregnancy. This is called Alpha-fetoprotein screening. This is a blood test that tests for neural tube defects or what is called Down Syndrome. It is important to have this type of testing done. Chances are the doctors will not find anything, however in case they do it is better to find out sooner rather than later.

You will also need to be tested for amniocentesis. This test is for chromosomal abnormalities. This test is also a test for Down Syndrome. This test is typically done in the first trimester.

There are various other blood tests that are done that test for abnormalities. Chromosomal abnormalities are the most common type of abnormalities that are found in new born babies. About 1 and every 150 babies have a chromosomal abnormality. Children that are born with chromosomal abnormalities have some sort of mental or birth defect.

The basic cause of chromosomal abnormality occurs when an error in the egg and the sperm occur.

Another unpleasant topic is miscarriages. They typically happen in the first 12 weeks of pregnancy if they happen. Miscarriages could happen in as many as 50% of all pregnancy's. However, only an estimated 15% of miscarriages are reported. Most women do not know that they are even pregnant until after they miscarry.

Chromosomal abnormalities and miscarriages are the reason why pregnant women should stay in constant contact with their doctors when they are pregnant.

The Postpartum Diet

One of the most important things to remember about the postpartum diet is that you will need between 300-500 more calories a day. Nursing the baby will take this many calories out of you, so it is important that you replace them.

The nurse feeding diet will require you to continue to keep a very healthy diet. The experts say it is best to basically maintain the same diet that you were eating when you were pregnant.

Below are the basic amounts of servings that your body will need when you are pregnant.

- Three servings of Protein are suggested

- Five servings of Calcium

- One or more servings of iron

- At least two servings of Vitamin C

- It is important to eat Green Foods

- Two servings of Fruits and Vegetables

- At least three servings of Carbohydrates

- Then it is important to get at least one serving of a high fat food

• Water intake is very important. At least eight glasses a day

It is important to continue to stay away from alcoholic beverages. When you are nursing it is important to stick with foods that your body knows. Do not try anything new. It is also best to stay away from any foods that you have had problems with in the past or that you know that you are allergenic too.

At this time it is also important to watch how much your baby is drinking if they are nursing from you. If they do not respond well after you ate something then it is probably best to stay away from that food. Give your baby what he or she wants when they are nursing from you. It is best to stay away from hot and spicy foods or anything that might upset the baby's stomach.

There is much debate as to how healthy breastfeeding still is. Many of the experts still agree that breastfeeding is the healthiest choice for both you are your baby. Breast feeding has many different positives and the positives outweigh the negatives. Here is a list of some of their many benefits.

• Breast feeding encourages a woman to eat healthy.

• A breastfeeding mother will lose weight because she is burning more calories.

• A baby that is breast fed will be less prone to illness.

• It is important that if you are breast feeding and taking medication that you be in consultation with the doctor to be sure that the medication that you are taking will not hurt the baby in any way.

It is also good to be aware of any toxins in the atmosphere when breast feeding. What I mean by this is to stay away from people that are smoking. Also it is not good to be in lawns that are freshly laid with pesticides. It is also good to stay away from people who have been sick.

Postpartum Depression

Postpartum depression is a common thing among young mothers. Postpartum depression is caused by many things. Here are a few things that might contribute to postpartum depression.

- The changes that pregnancy and delivery bring

- The social changes you face. Such as little time with friends.

- The lack of free time you once had

- Not getting enough sleep

- Anxiety about your ability to be a good mother

You might be more prone to postpartum depression if you are a mother that is very young. Also if this is your first pregnancy you could be more prone to be depressed than say it is your second or third pregnancy. If you have ever had trouble with a substance such as smoking or alcohol then you are a lot more prone to postpartum depression. If the pregnancy was not planned then you might also be more prone. Financial problems and maybe you broke up with the person you had the child with are also other huge reasons for postpartum depression.

A few of the symptoms that are struggling with post-partum depression are as follows.

• If you are always irritable

• Many appetite changes

• If you have a low self-esteem

• If you feel like you are not connected

• If you struggle with low energy levels

• If you struggle with a lot of anxiety

• If you have trouble sleeping at night

Mothers who struggle with severe postpartum depression might even be afraid to be alone with their baby. It is also not totally unheard of for a mother with severe postpartum depression to think about harming her baby. If this is ever the case the mother needs to seek professional help.

Some health care professionals recommend that a woman eat fish to help avoid postpartum depression. Why this is, is because of the omega-3 fatty acids found in the fish. The omega oils can help a woman avoid depression. It is also suggested to avoid the mercury that might be found in fish that just taking supplements that have omega fatty acids. This could greatly reduce the chances of struggling with severe depression after she gives birth to her first newborn. In most cases eating a healthy diet will also avoid the chances of having severe postpartum depression.

It is estimated that about 10% of women will struggle with some sort of postpartum depression.

Conclusion

Staying healthy when you are pregnant is very important. It is important to actually be healthy long before you even get pregnant. A healthy mother will produce a baby that is full of health and life.

There are many aspects that go into staying healthy when you are pregnant. It is not only your physical health, but also your emotional health that is important when you are pregnant. If you are emotionally healthy then it is very likely that you will be physically healthy as well.

It is important that you when you are pregnant to eat a lot of fruits and vegetables. Get the proper amount of protein in your diet. Drinking dairy products is also very important. You will need a lot of extra calcium so that the baby's bones and teeth grow properly. Remember it is best to eat six meals a day when you are pregnant. This includes eating a lot of very healthy snacks as meals. You need to be sure that all food that you are eating has been prepared in a safe atmosphere. Also stay away from all raw foods. This includes raw seafood such as sushi.

During your pregnancy it is important to get plenty of exercise. The best type of exercise a pregnant woman can do is to walk. It is important to stay away from weights and if you do insist on lifting weights when pregnant be sure to have someone around who can help you. Even when someone is around to help you it is best to not lift weights over your head.

Be sure to stay away from toxic environments. Stay away from lawns that have just been sprayed with insect-icide. Stay away from people who smoke.

Be sure to stay peaceful when you are pregnant. The baby will be able to tell if you are anxious or nervous. For your own health as well as the baby's health stay as calm as you possibly can throughout your entire pregnancy.

To conclude, have a great pregnancy! Stay healthy and everything will be fine.

About The Author

Becky Flynn is a writer living in Madison Wisconsin. She is currently at work on: "Nutritious Diet Durning Pregnancy: A Must For Delivering A Healthy Birth Weight Baby" among other titles.